B VITAMINS AND MENTAL HEALTH

B VITAMINS AND MENTAL HEALTH

Thank you for your continued support:

Facebook:
https://www.facebook.com/drgilliamlovesnaturalsolutions?ref=bookmarks

Email: drtiffany.gilliam@gmail.com

Dr. Tiffany Gilliam, N.D., MH, CNC, CHS

Copyright © 2015 by Dr. Tiffany Gilliam, N.D., MH, CNC, CHS

All rights reserved. This book or any portion thereof

may not be reproduced or used in any manner whatsoever

without the express written permission of the publisher

except for the use of brief quotations in a book review.

Printed in the United States of America

First Printing, 2015

All rights reserved.

ISBN-13: 978-1522721277

ISBN-10: 1522721274

DISCLAIMER

Although the author and publisher have made every effort to ensure that the information in this book was correct at press time, the author and publisher do not assume and hereby disclaim any liability to any party for any loss, damage, or disruptions caused by errors or omissions, whether such errors or omissions result from the negligence, accident or any other cause.

This book is not intended as a substitute for the medical advice of physicians. The reader should regularly consult a physician in matters relating to his/her health and particularly with respect to any symptoms that may require diagnosis or medical attention.

This is a reference tool with information to assist readers and practitioners with information and strategy that you opt is the best for you and your situation, circumstance, and condition.

The authors and affiliate parties are not responsible for individual choices and not to be held liable in any way, shape or form, based on any of the information gathered and/or followed by anyone.

CONTENTS

Chapter 1	1
<u>1.</u> Introduction	1
1.1. Vitamin B	1
1.2 Types of Vitamin B	2
1.2.1 Vitamin B1 or Thiamine	2
1.2.2. Vitamin B2 or Riboflavin	4
1.2.3. Vitamin B3 or Niacin	5
1.2.4. Vitamin B5 or Pantothenic acid	7
1.2.5. Vitamin B6 or Pyridoxal 5'-phosphate	9
1.2.6. Vitamin B7 or Biotin	10
1.2.7. Vitamin B9 or Folic Acid	12
1.2.8. Vitamin B12 or Cobalamin	13
1.3. Molecular Function	14
1.3.1. Vitamin B1 (Thiamine)	14
1.3.2. Vitamin B2 (Riboflavin)	15
1.3.3. Vitamin B3 (Niacin)	16
1.3.4. Vitamin B5 (Pantothenic acid)	17
1.3.5. Vitamin B6 (Pyridoxine, Pyridoxamine, and Pyridoxal)	18
1.3.6. Vitamin B7 (Biotin)	19

1.3.7. Vitamin B9	20
1.3.8. Vitamin B12	20
1.4. Aims and Objectives	21
Chapter 2	22
2. The B Vitamins and mental health	22
2.1. Role of Vitamin B1 in mental health	22
2.1.1. Wernicke–Korsakoff Syndrome	23
2.1.2. Beriberi	26
2.2. Role of Vitamin B2 in Mental Health	27
2.3. Role of Vitamin B6 in Mental Health	30
2.4. Role of Vitamin B9 in Mental health	32
2.5. Role of Vitamin B12 in Mental health	34
Chapter 3	45
3. Literature Review	45
Chapter 4	62
4. Recommendations	62
Chapter 5	64
5. Conclusion	65
Chapter 6	67
6. References	67

Chapter 1

1. Introduction

1.1. Vitamin B

Vitamins are a class of naturally occurring chemical compounds needed in fixed amounts for important body functions. They play important roles in energy generations, red blood cells and neurochemical production. They are micro-nutrients which are involved in the biological wear and tear of the body and an important part of a balance diet. Since the human body cannot produce vitamins which are required in normal concentration; they can be gained either from food sources or from dietary supplements. There are total of 13 kinds of vitamins needed by the human body comprising of vitamin A, vitamin C, vitamin D, vitamin K, and eight included in the group vitamin B (B1, B2, B3, B5, B6, B7, B9, and B12). Vitamin B group or complex contains all the water soluble vitamins that play an important role in metabolism. Due to the watery composition of our body, these vitamins have the ability to move inside our body and can be removed through urine without any difficulty. Thus, such vitamins are not stored by our bodies and need replenishing on a daily basis. Fruits and vegetables are rich sources of vitamin B complex for the body. Processed foods lose their vitamin B content through the process of enrichment as specified by food laws and regulations, the vitamin B is added into the food. Rich sources of vitamin B include potatoes, whole grains, legumes, nuts, meat and fish. Due to their delicate chemical nature, vitamin B complex is destroyed by excessive cooking and alcohol. Multiple processing of food reduces the nutritional content in the form of vitamin B complex. Vitamin B can be stored for limited time periods thus an improper diet can result in vitamin B deficiency just in a few months. Multiple tests are used to diagnose the vitamin B deficiency along with the help of different symptoms. Multiple symptoms linked with the vitamin B deficiency are dermatitis, numbness, anemia, insomnia, depression, amnesia, and fatigue. Multiple cases have been presented in which deficiency results from inadequacy of the body to absorb the required vitamin B from food sources. Following are the eight types of vitamin included in vitamin B complex:

1.2 Types of Vitamin B

1.2.1 Vitamin B1 or Thiamine

Vitamin B1 or thiamine is a sulfur containing vitamin required for converting glucose obtained from food into energy. It helps in energy production, normal appetite and maintenance of the nervous system. It is also found to be significant for electrolyte flow in the nerve cells thus regulating the functioning of the nervous system. Because of the important role of vitamin B1 in the metabolism of energy, reduced amount or deficiency can limit all of the vital functions of the body. Thiamine is used by all living organisms but their production is limited to plants, fungi and bacteria. Thiamine is found abundantly in pork, legumes, whole grains, fortified cereals and bread. As thiamine is present in the outer layer of grain which is usually removed in the refining thus refined and processed flour lose most of its thiamine content. Similarly the heat induced cooking methods and microwave treatments can also reduce the thiamine content in food by 20-50%. Other important sources of thiamine include cauliflower, liver, asparagus, brown rice, and potatoes.[1]

Most of the enzymes involved in cellular processes are dependent on thiamine for energy thus decreased in the intake of vitamin B1 affect the function of all cellular systems. As the nervous system and brain function is highly dependent on the oxidative metabolism, hence the nervous system gets highly affected by deficiency in thiamine level.

---

[1] Von Muralt 1958:72.

It specifically causes deterioration of peripheral nervous system, cerebellum and thalamus. Usually starting from muscle weakness and neurological confusion, if deficiency is persist it can lead to a coma and in adverse cases death as well.

1.2.2. Vitamin B2 or Riboflavin

Riboflavin is an important vitamin required for production of energy through metabolism of carbohydrates, proteins and fats, and through electron transport chains. It is also responsible for the activation of other vitamins by influencing the flavoprotein reactions. Its role is also established in the formation of RBCs, synthesis of niacin and stimulating good vision. Important sources of vitamin B2 are green vegetables, legumes, nuts, liver (meat, chicken and fish), cheese, and milk. Cereals are also a source of vitamin B2 but in very minimal quantity. The vitamin B2 is lost to great extent by the processing of cereals in mills. Different countries have introduced the enrichment process to add the required vitamin content after refining. Similarly, polished rice usually does not contain vitamin B2 as its yellow color will affect the appearance of polished rice. The vitamin B2 or riboflavin is not affected by the heat treatment of the food or during the cooking process. Deficiency in riboflavin levels can result in dermatitis on the lips and nose, cataract, red tongue, and light sensitivity. In multiple cases, the deficiency in riboflavin has also resulted in iron absorption and hemoglobin levels in blood thus adversely affecting the oxygen carrying capacity of red blood cells. The reduced rate of riboflavin in pregnant women can induce multiple developmental deformities in the fetus. Some studies also report different adverse effects of deficiency of Riboflavin in different cancers.[2]

1.2.3. Vitamin B3 or Niacin

Niacin is a general term used for all the compounds which resemble the activity of vitamin B3. Vitamin B3 contain group of enzyme pre-cursor compounds namely niacin, nicotinic acid, and nicotinamide. Niacin along with the nicotinamide acts as the precursor of enzymes, nicotinamide adenine dinucleotide phosphate (NADP) and nicotinamide adenine dinucleotide (NAD). Both of these enzymes are pivotal for the metabolic reactions as well as genetic repair and signaling mechanism. During different researches and test, vitamin B3 activity is measured through the level of nicotinamide. Vitamin B3 is also a great source of energy production through converting the food based protein, carbohydrate and fats content into energy products. Vitamin B3 is also a

---

[2] Spector, Maass, Michaud, Elvehjem & Hart 1943:75-87.

source of starch production that is then stored in the liver and muscle as energy storage. The energy is produced by vitamin B3 by slaking radicals which also provide protection against tissue damage. Niacin is also involved in genetic repair mechanism and secretion of hormones specifically steroids from adrenal glands. The role of niacin is also established in lowering the level of cholesterol in body thus niacin is usually prescribed to patients of high cholesterol and cardiac disorders.[3]

The food sources of vitamin B3 are chicken, tuna, turkey, legumes, nuts, vegetables, mushrooms, and grains like barley and brown rice. In the body, vitamin B3 or niacin can also be derived from tryptophan which is usually found in high protein food. The vitamin B3 based foods are stable with vitamin B3 remain intact during most of the processing. Extensive heating and boiling can result in the leeching out of the vitamin into water. Traditionally many cultures and communities, who rely on the corn as the source of vitamin, use cooking methods like post ash and lime water solution which preserves the maximum content of the food source. Deficiency of Vitamin B3 can result in anemia, lethargy, skin lesions, nausea and headaches. Deficiency is usually encountered in population

---

[3] Jacob & Swendseid, 1996:184-190.

with malnutrition or in low economic area. One of the distinguished deficiencies of vitamin B3 reported is pellagra. Pellagra is characterized by three D's symptoms: dementia, dermatitis, and diarrhea. Additional symptoms include hair loss, skin lesions, aggression, and insomnia. If pellagra is left untreated it can cause death within a period of five years. It is observed to be prevalent in alcoholic and malnutrition populations of Africa, China, Korea, and Indonesia.

1.2.4. Vitamin B5 or Pantothenic acid

Vitamin B5 which is also known as Pantothenic acid derive its name from Greek word (*pantos*) which mean everywhere thus its sources are widespread and found in all living organism. It belongs to the class of water soluble vitamins. Vitamin B5 help in converting the food ingested into a useable energy form, glucose. It also metabolizes the food component; carbohydrates, proteins and fats into an energy product to be utilized by the body. It is also involved in the synthesis of the red blood cells, neurotransmitters, and hormones. Pantothenic acid is involved in the production of acetyl coenzyme which transfers carbon atoms in the cell. Moreover, the pantothenic acid and acetyl coenzyme also play important role in synthesis of high energy compounds including acetylcholine, fatty acids, and cholesterol. Through affecting the production of multiple enzymes vitamin B5 has a role in signal transduction and activation and deactivation of enzymes in multiple metabolic pathways. Studies have indicated the role of vitamin B5 in reducing the cholesterol level in blood and in different cardiovascular disorders. The major sources of food are meat (specifically liver, brain and kidney), whole grains (rice and brain), vegetables like broccoli and avocados and seafood like cold water fish. In most of the food sources, vitamin B5 is present in the form of acyl carrier protein thus it is converted to pantothenic acid for absorption by body cells.[4]

Very rare cases of vitamin B5 deficiency has been reported as symptoms can easily be reversed upon diet improvement. The common symptoms are lethargy, depression, aggression, irritability, nausea, and respiratory tract infections. Due to deficiency in acetyl coenzyme A and acetylcholine, neurological disorders have also been observed in few cases. Symptoms usually occur in individuals already suffering from deficiency of vitamin B.

---

[4] Tahiliani & Beinlich 1990:165-228.

1.2.5. Vitamin B6 or Pyridoxal 5'-phosphate

Vitamin B6 is a group of compounds very similar in chemical structure and easily interconverted in system. In the natural system six active forms of Vitamin B6 exists namely pyridoxine (pyridoxol), pyridoxal, pyridoxamine, and phosphorylated forms of these three compounds. The vitamin B6 is an active cofactor of enzymes involved in the important pathway of glucose and amino acid metabolism. Vitamin B6 is an essential co enzyme for the enzyme required to produce glucose from glycogen in the body thus responsible for generating energy. It is also involved in the synthesis of neurotransmitters like serotonin, dopamine, glutamate, D-serine, and histamine. Similarly, the Pyridoxal 5'-phosphate is also involved in the synthesis of heme group of hemoglobin. Vitamin B6 has the ability to reduce the levels of homocysteine whose increased levels have been encountered in multiple cardiovascular diseases. Its role has recently been discovered in reducing depression in the late years of life.

Pyridoxal 5'-phosphate (PLP) is essential for the function of more than 100 enzymes of metabolic pathways though it cannot be produced with in the body and has to be obtained directly from the food. The daily intake of protein effects the level of vitamin B6 in the body. The food rich in proteins and vitamin B6 are whole grains, milk, eggs, meat, vegetables (including potatoes, spinach, peas and carrot), and legumes. Due to being water soluble, the vitamin B6 can be lost from the food through excess heating and processing of the food source. The vitamin B6 in plant sources are far more stable than animal sources as it is present usually in pyridoxine form in plants as compared to pyridoxal form in animals.

If the required amount of vitamin B6 is not ingested, it can adversely affect the major metabolic reactions of the body. In children, developing nervous systems get affected due to reduced levels of PLP in the body. Most common symptoms of vitamin B6 deficiency are skin sores, depression, lethargy, and irritability. Common syndromes reported with the deficiency of vitamin B6 are conjunctivitis, atrophic glossitis with ulceration, angular cheilitis, and neurologic symptoms of confusion, and neuropathy.

1.2.6. Vitamin B7 or Biotin

Vitamin B7 which is also known as Biotin and coenzyme R which is another water soluble vitamin. Biotin plays a significant role in the metabolic pathways of amino acids and fats as well as in the cell growth cycle. It is also required to keep the stable sugar level in the body. Biotin acts as an active coenzyme for the functional class of enzyme, carboxylases. Eight forms of biotin exist in nature but only D-biotin has the vitamin characteristics and activity. Although it is essential in all living organisms, it can only be produced in the body of plants, yeast, algae, bacteria and molds.

Biotin plays an important role in converting fat, proteins and carbohydrates into glucose to generate energy in the body. Vitamin B7 is also very important for the strength of hair and nails by activating metabolism process. The mucous membrane and skin development is maintained in the presence of biotin. By regulating different metabolic reaction, vitamin B7 is essential for psychological functions of the body.

The level of biotin is specifically monitored in the pregnancy but no studies have yet revealed the direct effect of biotin in the development of the fetus. The deficiency of vitamin B7 in body results in weakening of hair and nails, skin rashes, depression, hallucination, and weariness. As a result of biotin deficiency, a disposition of fats on facial area has also been observed. Children who develop vitamin B7 deficiency in earlier years have compromised immune systems and as a result frequently develop different infections.

Different food sources of vitamin B7 are raw egg yolk, Liver, meat, Whole grain, Avocado, soybeans and nuts.

1.2.7. Vitamin B9 or Folic Acid

Vitamin B9 which is also referred as folic acid, vitamin M and pteroyl-L-glutamate is also a water soluble vitamin. For the biological activity, it is to be converted into folate in the body. It is essential for the synthesis of nucleic acid in the body. It also helps in regulating the cell division, cell growth as well as production of new red blood cells in the body. Folic acid plays an important role in metabolism of nucleic acid as purines and thymidine uses folate as coenzyme to synthesize DNA. Folic acid also plays important role in controlling gene expression by regulating methylation process. Some studies have also indicated the probable role of folic acids in the mental health. The human body has no mechanism to store the folic acids in the body rather it has to be consumed on daily basis to fulfill its requirement.

Consumption of folic acid is very necessary for the pregnant woman as well as lactating mothers. It is required for the increased cell division, growth and energy requirement of the body. It helps in preventing different birth defects and enables normal brain and spinal development in the fetus. If during the pregnancy the deficiency of folic acid in body occurs, it can be translated into congenital and neural tube defects. The bone marrow cells are more prone to vitamin B9 deficiency due to their rapid division thus resulting in condition of megaloblastic anemia. Due to reduce amount of folate available to bone marrow cells, the formation of red blood cells is reduced causing the condition of anemia. Folate also reduces the risk of cardiovascular disorders by regulating the level of homocysteine in the body. Furthermore, studies have also indicated the role of folic acid in reducing the symptoms of depression. Common food sources of Folic acid are broccoli, cabbage, cauliflower, egg, liver, kidneys, spinach, peas, soybeans, asparagus and whole grains.

1.2.8. Vitamin B12 or Cobalamin

Among all the water soluble vitamins, Cobalamin or vitamin B12 has the most intricate structure as it contains the cobalt ion in its structure. In the body, the vitamin B12 is converted to methylcobalamin and 5-deoxyadenosylcobalamin to perform its function. Vitamin B12 is a coenzyme of important folate related enzyme methionine synthase which is required for the synthesis of methionine and amino acid. These enzymes are also important for the regulating the gene expression through methylation. Its role is also established in the synthesis of red blood cells. Due to deficiency of vitamin B12, the common symptoms observed are lethargy, headaches, nausea, lack of appetite, poor vision, psychosis, dementia, ulcers, and skin sores. Some studies have also indicated the role of Vitamin B12 deficiency in cognitive defect, peripheral neuropathy and Alzheimer's.

As bacteria are the only living organism who can synthesize the vitamin B12 thus it can be usually obtained from the animal sources like egg, milk, meat, fish and lesser quantities from plants like soybeans and rice.

1.3. Molecular Function

1.3.1. Vitamin B1 (Thiamine)

Vitamin B1 also referred to as thiamine is a group of water-soluble vitamins that plays a significant role in various chemical reactions of the body. It mainly helps the body's cells to convert carbohydrate into adenosine triphosphate (ATP), a chemical that is used for energy by the body's cells mainly brain and nervous system. Furthermore, thiamine keeps eyes, hair, skin and liver healthy. It strengthens the immune system. Thiamine is also responsible for the generation of DNA and RNA. During metabolism pyruvate is converted to acetyl coenzyme A by an active form of thiamine known as Thiamine pyrophosphate (TPP).[5]

---

[5] Cooper & Pincus 1979:223-239.

1.3.2. Vitamin B2 (Riboflavin)

Vitamin B2 also referred as Riboflavin helps in generating energy for the body's cells. It also acts as an antioxidant that works to wash out free radicals from the body. It performs an important role in converting folate and vitamin B6 into usable forms. Furthermore, it helps in the red blood cell production in the body. When Riboflavin is active in the body's energy pathways it changes itself into Flavin adenine dinucleotide (FAD) or Flavin mononucleotide (FMN) and then attaches itself to protein enzymes and allows oxygen-based energy production. FMN and FAD when attach to proteins are called as flavoproteins that can be found all over the body especially at sites where oxygen-based energy production is demanded.[6]

Furthermore, Flavin mononucleotide (FMN) and Flavin adenine dinucleotide (FAD) act as cofactor in various flavoprotein enzyme reactions. One of the important role it plays is as a cofactor of methylenetetrahydrofolate reductase (MTHFR) which is important in the degradation of excess homocysteine which is associated with the risk of heart disease.

---

[6] Ball 2008.

Numerous metabolic and energy production processes in the body demand oxygen. Molecules having oxygen are highly reactive and harmful to the tissues and blood vessels present in the body. In order to protect the damage another small protein like molecule named glutathione is produced. However, constant recycling of glutathione is mandatory in order convert it back to its reduced form. Enzyme glutathione reductase in the presence of vitamin B2 as co-factor helps in recycling glutathione.

1.3.3. Vitamin B3 (Niacin)

Vitamin B3 also referred to as niacin is responsible for the production of energy in the body by the conversion of food into glucose. Nicotinamide is an active form of niacin which is a precursor to two coenzymes nicotinamide adenine dinucleotide phosphate (NADP) and nicotinamide adenine dinucleotide (NAD). NAD and NADP help in the activation of various dehydrogenases participating in electron transport chain and in other cellular respiratory reactions. NAD contributes mainly in catabolic reactions such as in the breakdown of fats, proteins and carbohydrates. It also facilitates DNA repair mechanism. On the other hand, NADP is important for anabolic reactions such as in the production of macromolecules such as cholesterol and fatty acids and also in steroid synthesis. The proper consumption of vitamin B3 in dietary intake is important for the maintenance of skin health along with the normal functioning of nervous and digestive system.[7]

1.3.4. Vitamin B5 (Pantothenic acid)

Vitamin B5 also referred to as pantothenic acid is responsible for making an important coenzyme *i.e.* coenzyme A in the body. Coenzyme A is involved in various biochemical reactions such as in the oxidation of carbohydrates, fatty acids and in the synthesis of steroid hormones, amino acids, cholesterol etc. Vitamin B5 is also used in the formation of acyl carrier proteins (ACP) which participates in the transformation of fatty acids into further complex molecules.[8]

1.3.5. Vitamin B6 (Pyridoxine, Pyridoxamine, and Pyridoxal)

Vitamin B6 is a part of vitamin B complex group which play their role in various biological functions. The active form of vitamin B6 is known as Pyridoxal 5'-phosphate (PLP) that serves as a cofactor in many enzyme reactions mainly in glucose, lipid and amino acid metabolism. Furthermore, it is involved in many aspects of macronutrient metabolism

---

[7] Sauve 2008:883-893.

[8] Noveup 1953.

such as histamine synthesis, neurotransmitter synthesis, hemoglobin function and synthesis, and gene expression. It also acts as a coenzyme in many chemical reactions including transamination, decarboxylation, racemization, replacement, elimination and beta-group interconversion. Metabolism of Vitamin B6 takes place in liver.

Vitamin B6 is crucial to the metabolism of sugar, starch and glycogen present in the body. It is important during pregnancy and infancy to help in the brain development. Furthermore, it also plays a vital role in the body's immune function. Vitamin B6 also has great and varied impact on nervous system. It aids in the development of amines also referred as message molecules or neurotransmitters which help in the transmission of messages from one nerve to another. Therefore, vitamin B6 also regulates moods and it plays a role in the creation of amine-derived neurotransmitters including, serotonin, epinephrine, norepinephrine and melatonin.

1.3.6. Vitamin B7 (Biotin)

Vitamin B7 is a water soluble B vitamin also referred to as biotin, vitamin H or coenzyme R. Vitamin B7 is involved in various digestive and metabolic processes. It attaches itself to five mammalian enzymes known as carboxylases. When a biotin molecular attaches a protein it is known as biotinylation. The biotinylation of apocarboxylases and histones is catalyzed by holocarboxylase synthetase. Furthermore, biotinidase catalyzes the release of biotin from the peptide products of carboxylase breakdown and from histones.

Each carboxylase having biotin attached as a cofactor catalyzes different essential metabolic reaction. For instance, acetyl- CoA carboxylase I and II catalyze the binding of acetyl- CoA to bicarbonate for the formation of malonyl- CoA required for the synthesis of fatty acids. Pyruvate carboxylase is another important enzyme that is involved in gluconeogenesis. Methylcrotonyl- CoA carboxylase is involved in an essential step in the catabolism of leucine. Porpionyl- CoA carboxylase is essential in catalyzing the metabolism of cholesterol, odd chain fatty acids and certain amino acids.

1.3.7. Vitamin B9

Vitamin B9 is also known as vitamin M or folic acid. It is an important component in our diet that must be obtained from food. It plays a vital role in a number of biochemical processes in a human body. Folate molecules produced from folic acid are involved in the transfer of one-carbon units in a number of reactions that are crucial to the metabolism of nucleic acids and amino acids. Therefore synthesis of DNA from its precursors depends on the presence of folate molecules as co-enzymes. These molecules also help prevent the mutation in DNA molecules that may result in the development of cancers. Folate molecules also help in the prevention of homocysteine accumulation that is a precursor of methionine and a contributor towards heart disease.

1.3.8. Vitamin B12

Vitamin B12 also known as cobalamin plays a vital role in the metabolism of folate and in the synthesis of succinyl-CoA, an intermediate of citric acid cycle. It also acts as a cofactor for methionine synthase, an enzyme required for the synthesis of methionine from homocysteine. Amino acids methionine is crucial for the synthesis of S-adenosylmethionine which is used in various biological methylation reactions.

Furthermore, vitamin B12 also acts as a cofactor for L-methylmalonyl-coenzyme A mutase which is further converted to succinyl-coenzyme A. This enzyme then enters the citric acid cycle and plays its role in the production of energy from proteins and lipids. Furthermore, it is also required in the formation of oxygen-carrying pigment in red blood cells known as hemoglobin.

1.4. Aims and Objectives

The present study aims at highlighting the role of vitamin B group in normal body functions and in crucial metabolic pathways for the wholeness of man. Molecular function of B vitamins is discussed in detail which is further linked to its role in mental health. Mental illness is commonly caused by the deficiency in the amount of vitamin B in the human body. Several serious disorders such as Wernicke-Korsakoff syndrome, schizophrenia, depression and anxiety are commonly linked with the deficiency of vitamin B. The current study discusses the role of vitamin B in causing mental illness, moreover recommendations are discussed so as to reduce the mortality and morbidity rate associated with the vitamin B group.

Chapter 2

2. The B Vitamins and mental health

2.1. Role of Vitamin B1 in mental health

Vitamin B1 is one of the eight vitamins of the powerful group known as vitamin B complex. It plays a vital role in maintaining sound mental health. It should be taken with great care as improper care and over dosage is harmful for the body. The main function of vitamin B1 is glucose metabolism. It converts carbohydrates to energy which is required for various metabolic activities of the body. Furthermore it aids in the normal functioning of nervous system, heart and musculature system of the body. Vitamin B is vital to particular areas of brain mainly the emotional health, focus and concentration. The need of vitamin B1 also known as thiamine increases during pregnancy, lactation and high fever. Its absorption is impaired by shellfish, tea and coffee. Severe deficiency of vitamin B1 results in beriberi, Korsakoff's psychosis and Wernicke's encephalopathy. Some people also experience confusion and disorientation which happens as a result of brain's inability for oxidizing glucose for energy as because the crucial cofactor involved in glycolysis and tricarboxylic acid is missing.

2.1.1. Wernicke–Korsakoff Syndrome

Wernicke–Korsakoff Syndrome is a brain disorder that is caused by the severe deficiency of vitamin B1. The disorder has two separate conditions that occur simultaneously. Initially the patient suffers from Wernicke's encephalopathy that causes bleeding in the lower areas of the brain mainly hypothalamus and thalamus that control endocrine and nervous systems. These areas are damaged by the bleeding that results in poor vision, balance and coordination. Later on, when Wernicke's symptoms diminish then the signs of Korsakoff psychosis begin. However, if Wernicke's disease is treated on time then more chances are that Korsakoff syndrome does not develop.

Korsakoff syndrome causes chronic brain damage and affects the regions of brain that control memory. The main cause associated with Wernicke-Korsakoff syndrome is malnutrition that results in the severe deficiency of thiamine (vitamin B1) in the body. Another important factor responsible for the syndrome is chronic alcoholism. Alcohol interferes with active gastrointestinal transport that decreases the activation of thiamine pyrophosphate from thiamine. Furthermore, chronic liver disease causes decreased capacity of liver to store thiamine. Individuals suffering from schizophrenia, terminal cancer, and anorexia nervosa are at risk of developing thiamine deficiency due to starvation. Studies have reported forty-nine cases of Wernicke encephalopathy in women going through pregnancy. People suffering from gastric malignancy and intestinal obstruction are also at high risk of developing the syndrome. It also occurs after plastic surgery and bariatric surgery and prevails if not treated timely. Moreover, people having systemic diseases such as acquired immunodeficiency syndrome (AIDS), uremia and malignancy disseminated tuberculosis may develop Wernicke-Korsakoff syndrome.

The syndrome has a complex pathophysiology. Vitamin B1 is absorbed in the body from duodenum. The body stores thiamine enough for eighteen days which is regularly converted into its active form known as thiamine pyrophosphate in the glial and neural cells. The active form of thiamine acts as cofactor in the functioning of several enzymes such as pyruvate dehydrogenase, transketolase, and alpha ketoglutarate which helps in the usage of glucose. The main role of these enzymes is carbohydrate and lipid metabolism in the brain. In addition to this these, the enzymes also produce amino acids and glucose derived neurotransmitters. Vitamin B1 has its role in the axonal conduction mainly in serotoninergic and acetylcholinergic neurons. Any kind of deficiency in the availability of these enzymes will result in loss of glucose metabolism in the keys areas of the brain that eventually results in impaired cellular energy metabolism. After continuous decrease in the levels of thiamine, the areas of the brain that require high thiamine levels start showing signs of injury and cellular impairment. Initially the activity of alpha-ketoglutarate dehydrogenase decreases in astrocytes. Severe vitamin B1 deficiency causes mitochondrial dysfunction that poisons the high metabolic areas of brain. Additional studies have also reported an extracellular glutamate concentrations, increased astrocyte lactate and edema, deoxyribonucleic acid fragmentation in neurons, increase in cytokines, increased astrocyte lactate and edema and breakdown of blood brain barrier. Vitamin B1 also appears to have role in axonal conduction, acetylcholinergic, and serotoninergic synaptic transmission. Wernicke-Korsakoff syndrome symptoms are mainly associated to these focal areas of damage. Lesions in the brainstem affect ocular motor signs which further affect the abducens nuclei and eye movement areas in the midbrain and pons. These lesions are mainly described by lack of significant destruction of nerve cells.

Cerebellum damage results in ataxia. These changes affect all the layers of the cortex mainly the Purkinje cells. Neuron loss causes serious ataxia of gait and stance. Along with the cerebellar dysfunction the vestibular apparatus is also affected. Moreover, excessive alcohol consumption leads to thirty-five percent reduction in transketolase activity in the cerebellum that is because of thiamine deficiency.

In the early stages of the disease, vestibular paresis is also confirmed but gets better with advancement of treatment. The memory loss or amnestic component is mainly associated with the damage in the diencephalon in addition with the medial thalamus and connections with amygdala and medial temporal lobes. Amnesia is irreversible structural damage and may not improve with treatment.

2.1.2. Beriberi

Beriberi also referred to as thiamine deficiency is caused mainly due to the lack of thiamine pyrophosphate, an active form of thiamine (Vitamin B1). Thiamine pyrophosphate acts as a cofactor in carbohydrate metabolism and participates in glucose formation by acting as a cofactor in the glucose metabolism pathway. Thiamine is absorbed in small intestine through an active transport portal and is then phosphorylated. Thiamine is not naturally produced by the body and is therefore stores in tissues. It is mainly found in skeletal muscles, brain, liver, heart and kidneys. Beriberi results from malnutrition, hyperthyroidism, lactation, fever and pregnancy.

Beriberi is mainly divided into two categories namely wet beriberi and dry beriberi. Wet beriberi is thiamine deficiency that damages heart, whereas dry beriberi effects nervous system. Malnutrition and physical inactivity contribute widely to the disease. The main problems as a result are peripheral neuropathy in which the sensory, motor and reflex functions are effected.

2.2. Role of Vitamin B2 in Mental Health

Vitamin B2 or riboflavin is one of the important water soluble vitamins that have significant role in regulating the nervous system as well as multiple metabolic reactions. In neurological system, the vitamin B2 is very important for the synthesis of monoamine, regulation of methylation process and oxidative reaction. The required level of vitamin B2 is very essential to synthesize the important enzyme L-methylfolate and converting the vitamin B6 in utilizable form in one carbon metabolism cycle. Multiple studies have investigated the role of riboflavin in decreasing the depressions, migraines and improving the cognition process. Depression and headaches are common symptoms of deficiency of riboflavin in the body. Riboflavin deficiency is very common in patients suffering from mild to severe depression and improvement has been observed to great extent after taking riboflavin as a supplement. The condition of depression as a result of deficiency of vitamin B2 is even more severe in alcoholic patients. In alcohol addicts, the major source of calories and energy is sugars in alcohol drinks that reduce the vitamin content in the body to great extent. Thus most of the alcohol addict suffers from vitamin deficiency which results in high prevalence of depression and related symptoms in alcohol consumers.

Upon entering the energy generation pathway, riboflavin is converted into Flavin mononucleotide FMN or in other words Flavin adenine dinucleotide FAD. FAD is an important cofactor molecule of an enzyme methylenetetrahydrofolate reductase (MTHFR) which have significant role in the metabolism of homocysteine on one carbon metabolism. Due to decreased activity of FAD or MTHFR, the level of homocysteine started to increase in brain tissue resulting in neurotoxicity, depression and a number of other neurological symptoms. The role of vitamin B is also established in the synthesis of glutathione which act as an antioxidant agent, detoxifying the toxic molecules in brain cells as well as in other parts of the body. Decreased levels of vitamin B2 is also believed to be associated with elevated level of toxins in the brain cells thus resulting in depression and other neurological symptoms.

Riboflavin is also used as a curative agent for migraine pain. Riboflavin not only reduces the amount of pain but also increase the occurrence duration of the migraine attacks. Riboflavin is prescribed in high doses to reduce the pain as well as preventive measure for migraine patients. The use of riboflavin has the capability to reduce the occurrence of migraine attacks actual mechanism by half in patients. The actual mechanism is not yet completely discovered but reduction in the pain of migraine is considered to be effect of improved availability of the energy for brain cells.

Deficiency of riboflavin is not very common because in developed country the vitamin is added in the food after processing. But the deficiency of vitamin B2 has been considered a risk factor for multiple nervous disorders such as numbness, Alzheimer's disease, anxiety, sclerosis and in few cases of epilepsy as well. The basic purpose of the vitamin B2 is to provide energy to the different cells of the body for proper functioning, the deficiency in the vitamin causes the gap between the energy demand and supply resulting in the shutting down of the function. The nervous system disorders discussed above results from the decreased energy supply due to deficiency in vitamin levels.

2.3. Role of Vitamin B6 in Mental Health

Vitamin B6 plays vital role in both physical and mental health. It is needed for proper absorption of vitamin B12. It functions as an essential coenzyme in the metabolism of fats, carbohydrates, and proteins. It is crucial for the formation of antibodies and red blood cells. It serves as an important coenzyme during metabolism of amino acids and nervous system. In the central nervous system, vitamin B6 aids the production of gamma-Amino butyric acid. Furthermore, vitamin B6 converts arachidonic acid to prostaglandin E2 and tryptophan to niacin.

Neurotransmitters acetylcholine and norepinephrine and histamine depend on the active form of vitamin B6 known as P5P. The brain requires vitamin B6 for converting tryptophan to serotonin. Studies have reported that vitamin B6 contributes to the proper functioning of over hundred enzymes. For instance, vitamin B6 and zinc are demanded for the production of hydrochloric acid and pancreatic enzymes. Furthermore, the combination of vitamin B6 and zinc is also needed for the creation of serotonin and other neurotransmitters in brain. These neurotransmitters play an important role in the communication of brain and nerve cells. This communication is to ensure that all the metabolic processes are running smoothly. Furthermore, it also solves a number of problems including premenstrual syndrome (PMS), nerve compression injuries, arthritis and depression conditions. It is also used in combination with vitamin B9 and vitamin B12 to treat high homocysteine levels. Moreover, vitamin B6 supplementation helps in treating diabetes, memory loss, kidney stones, lung cancer, atherosclerosis, and attention deficit-hyperactivity disorder (ADHD).

The central nervous system essentially needs an adequate supply of glucose and all the essential nutrients for a healthy brain function. Vitamin B6 along with vitamin B9 and vitamin B12 participate in one-carbon metabolism, a pathway vital for healthy brain function. Therefore, deficiency in any of the enzymes involved in the pathway is related with severe damage of brain function. One-carbon metabolism pathway is characterized by the generation of one-carbon units with the help of serine that is activated through association with tetrahydrofolate. The product 5, 10- methylenetetrahydrofolate is further used for the formation of purines, thymidylate, and methionine. Purines and thymidylate play their part in nucleic acid synthesis and methionine is crucial for biological methylations and protein synthesis. Various studies have reported that methionine synthesis pathway is vital in maintaining the health of brain tissue.

2.4. Role of Vitamin B9 in Mental health

Vitamin B9 also referred to as folate is a vital coenzyme that aids the synthesis of genetic material (DNA). It also plays a crucial role in cellular development, growth, function, and reproduction. Folic acid promotes a healthy pregnancy as it controls the development of fetus nervous system. It is a critical vitamin that has its role in every growth phases of human life.

In one-carbon metabolism, folic acid and vitamin B12 act as co-enzymes. A glycine and serine carbon unit react with tetrahydrofolate (THF) to produce methylene-THF which is further employed in the synthesis of thymidylate (DNA nucleotide) or purine. Macrotic anemia is a result of folate deficiency caused by mainly the failure of blood cell division because of the lack of DNA. Methionine synthase (MS) catalyzes the re-methylation of homocysteine to methionine in the presence of vitamin B12 that acts a cofactor. If methionine synthase gets deactivated due to deficiency of vitamin B12 than as a result functional folate deficiency occurs as folate remains trapped as methyl-THF. Another consequence of folate and vitamin B12 deficiency is hyperhomocysteinemia.[9]

Dietary folate is hydrolyzed in the intestine and is fully methylated and reduced to form 5-methyltetrahydrofolate which aids the transport within body including blood brain barrier and through cell membrane. High concentrations of folate reside in the brain and in cerebrospinal fluid

---
[9] Selhub, Morris, Jacques & Rosenberg 2009:702S-706S.

that is 17-41 µg/l which is thrice the amount found in blood. Vitamins are not normally allowed to pass through blood brain barrier instead particular active transport systems are used to transport vitamins across the blood brain barrier. Methylation is a crucial phenomenon in the central nervous system as it modulates DNA methylation which is critical in development. Furthermore, folate also improves the storage of a metabolic precursor of coenzyme A, pantothenic acid which is an important compound to nervous system. Folate deficiency also has a role in congenital anomalies. The babies of the mothers having low levels of folate have neural tube defects. However, folate supplementation reduces the risk of such serious birth problems.

Studies have proved that mental illness is never caused by a single factor alone but many medical conditions along with certain genes cause mental illness. Individuals suffering from mental illness are at increased risk of vitamin deficiencies. Similarly low levels of folate are associated with dementia and depression. Studies have reported folate as an effective remedy for treatment of depression. Folate also has positive effect on the aging of the brain. The role of vitamin B12 in Mental Health.

2.5. Role of Vitamin B12 in Mental health

Vitamin B12 or Cobalamin is an important cofactor that plays an important role in one-carbon cycle and is required for the production and metabolism of neurotransmitters. Vitamin B12 also maintains the level of myelin in the body. The decreased level of vitamin B12 can result in psychosis, irritability, depression, compulsive symptoms, and Alzheimer's disease. The one carbon cycle is a metabolic reaction in which transfer of carbon unit take place from glycine or serine to tetrahydrofolate from the product methylene-tetrahydrofolate. This product tetrahydrofolate has multiple uses in the body; it is used for the production of one of the DNA building block thymidine, for the production of purines after oxidation, and to convert methylate homocysteine to methionine after reduction. The methionine synthesized in the presence of vitamin B12 is further converted to a methyl group donor, S-adenosylmethionine (SAM) which causes the methylation and activation of neurotransmitters, hormones, proteins, membrane lipids, DNA, and RNA. Without the successful methylation, above mentioned molecule remain inactive and is not read by the transcription and translation machinery of the body. Due to this important role of vitamin B12 in methylation, activation and synthesis of neurotransmitters, special attention has been given to the relation of vitamin B12 levels in the body and neurological diseases like Alzheimer's disease and the loss of neurological cognitive function.

Another mechanism of onset of these neurological problems has been associated with elevated levels of homocysteine. In the deficiency of vitamin B12 in the body the precursor molecule of methionine, homocysteine started to increase as enough vitamin B12 is not present to convert it into methionine. High levels of homocysteine results in neurotoxicity in the brain cells as well as high numbers of hypomethylated neurological tissues. The hypomethylation has been established as a major cause of Alzheimer's disease, reduce cognitive function and increase tendency of developing depression.

Reduced levels of vitamin B12 in the body can result in damaging the protective sheath of nerves known as myelin. Without the protective myelin sheath, the nerves fail to perform proper function thus resulting in impairment of the nervous system. The degeneration of myelin resulted from deficient level of vitamin B12 caused nerve damage and spinal cord degeneration. Similarly, vitamin B12 or cobalamin is required for the synthesis of succinyl Coenzyme A from the precursor, methylmelonyl Coenzyme A. In the absence or reduced levels of vitamin B12, the methymelonyl CoA is transformed into another product known as methylmalonic acid which is established destabilizer agent of myelin. If the deficiency of vitamin B12 persist, it can result in an elevated level of methylmalonic acid which in turn will cause the formation of deformed fatty acids in place of normal myelin. Due to a deformed fatty acid compound, the protective sheath formed on nerves is fragile and insubstantial known as demyelination. The demyelination process can result in impairment of the central nervous system as well as peripheral nervous system.

Sub-acute combined spinal cord degeneration is a common outcome of demyelination due to vitamin B12 deficiency. It is also referred in multiple studies as Lichtheim disease and is characterized by the degeneration of lateral and posterior columns of the peripheral nervous system. The onset of the disease is caused by complete loss of myelin sheath in the lateral and dorsal columns. Due to nerve impairment, patients encounter the feeling of numbness and weakening of arms and legs and in some cases patients also experience vision impairment. If the vitamin B12 deficiency persists, the sense of touch starts to deteriorate and prolonged period of condition causes permanent damage to the nervous system. The common symptoms of condition are loss in recognition and sense of temperature, pain and touch, numbness, abnormal reflexes, erectile dysfunction, and impaired cognition.

Psychosis-Another important neurological disorder associated with the deficiency of vitamin B12 is known as psychosis in which normal cognition process is impaired to an extent that person lack the ability to distinguish the reality from hallucinations and imaginations. Disease is also linked with mobility issues and social withdrawal and isolation symptom which can also cause the onset of depression in patients. The prolonged condition of psychosis poses a threat to the safety of patient as self-harm is common outcome of advance psychosis. Different types of psychosis exist including the reactive psychosis, drug related psychosis and organic psychosis. The reactive psychosis is a result of a stressful and traumatic event which act as a trigger for the psychosis condition. But this type of psychosis is short lived and usually patients came out of the condition with treatment. Drug or alcohol related psychosis occur due to excessive use of alcohol and other drugs. These drugs not only increase the amount of neurotoxins but also reduce the amount of Vitamin B12 resulting in increased neurotoxicity in nervous system and reduced antioxidant activity thus causing hallucinations and imaginations. Organic psychosis is the result of onset of condition due to brain injury or other neurological illness that may or may not have arisen from the deficiency of vitamin B12.

Dementia- also referred as memory loss is a condition of mental deterioration which may occur due to degeneration of nerve cells, neurotransmitters and axon damage. It is a progressive condition and limits the normal functioning of the brain. The initial symptoms comprise of memory loss to an extent that restrict the functioning. The memory loss is followed by onset of anxiety and depression. Dementia also effects the coordination and balance of the body with changes in behavior and mood. With the progress of the condition, patients losses the ability to communicate and interpret the environment around him/her. Delusion, imaginations and hallucinations are also common symptoms of dementia. In the MRI scans of the dementia patients, the brain size is observed to decrease which is correlated with the decrease amount of vitamin B12 in the body. In many elderly patients, the condition of dementia and other neurological disorders have resulted not from the deficiency of vitamin B12 in body but reduction in the ability to absorb the vitamin B12 from food. The digestion of vitamin B12 is a complex process and requires a set of proteins which break the bond between protein content and vitamin B12 content of the food. Though enough amount of vitamin B12 is ingested but body fails to utilize this vitamin B12 for the brain cell development its result dementia, Alzheimer's and other neurological disorders. As the absorption and digestion of vitamin B12 deteriorate with age thus most of the neurological disorders are observed in advance age. The ability of brain cells to form connections resulting in memory is possible due to vitamin B12, similarly the importance of cobalamin for the protection of brain cells in the form of myelin is an established fact. Another cause of dementia is the condition of pernicious anemia which also arises from the deficiency of vitamin B12. The condition of pernicious anemia arises when the bone marrow starts to produce red blood cells that are larger in size and less in numbers. This condition arises from the inability to absorb the required vitamin B12 from food.

Alzheimer's disease-is a neurological degenerative disorder this is characterized by condition of dementia and behavioral issue. The Alzheimer's initial symptoms are memory lapses and memory loss but as condition progresses with age the memory loss is further accompanied by disorientation, behavioral issues, and depression. Gradually the mental health deterioration is followed by the loss of bodily functions and eventually death. Though the factors responsible for the onset of disease are still understudy and include from genetic to physiological causes.

Role of vitamin B12 in disease onset is recently been established and studies are being conducted to provide evidence for this relation. As in most of the patients, the brain size is reduced which is correlated to the deficiency of vitamin B12. The onset of disease is split into four stages: Pre-dementia, before the clinical detection of the Alzheimer's disease, patient often develops symptoms of cognitive impairment and short term memory loss. These symptoms are usually associated with advancing age thus patients usually ignore the need of medical assistance. Early depression and irritability is encountered commonly in this stage. Patients starting to experience difficulty in cognitive activities like attentiveness, planning, and concentration. With progression of disease, the earlier symptoms started to appear including the memory loss and learning impairment which is referred to as the early phase of the disease. The memory issues are followed by behavioral problems including perceptions, confusion, and increased irritability. Patients also experience difficulty in communication because of the limited vocabulary and fluency. As the disease continue to progress and enter into moderate stage, the difficulty increases in the daily activities with increased inability to communicate, remembering details and comprehending ideas. In this stage along with the short- term memory the long-term memory also starts to deteriorate. The final stage of the disease is characterized by extreme memory loss, complete dependability, emotional aggression, irritability, and reduces mobility. The direct association of vitamin B12 level with the Alzheimer's is under study but many researchers believe that elevated level of homocysteine is responsible for the onset of Alzheimer's as a result of vitamin B12 deficiency.

Peripheral neuropathy is also very common neurological disturbance that arises due to vitamin B12 deficiency. In peripheral neuropathy, the communication mechanism between the part of the body and spinal cord is affected due to improper nerve signal transmission. This may arise due to the weakening of myelin sheath and axon damage due to reduce level of vitamin B12 in the body. Due to peripheral nerve damage, muscle activity also gets affected resulting in local immobility, muscle impairment, and loss of organ function. It can cause muscle loss, cramps, convulsing, and even bone degeneration in some cases. If the peripheral neuropathy occurs in motor nerves, it can result in loss of coordination and balance, known as motor neuropathy. The demyelination in the sensory neurons can result into loss of senses of touch, temperature and pain and also cause coordination problems known as sensory neuropathy. Another form of peripheral neuropathy is autonomic neuropathy that affects the function of different organs and glands.

Increase in homocysteine levels causes the brain shrinkage which is known as atrophy. The brain shrinkage is a normal process that occurs with advancing age but due to deficiency of vitamin B12 the atrophy rate increases resulting in onset of multiple neurological disorders. The reduced level of Vitamin B12 has been encountered in Parkinson disease, Alzheimer's and dementia.

During fetal development, the vitamin B12 is stored in fetal liver that can be used month after the birth. But most of the children are prone to deficiency of vitamin B12 from age of 6 months to 12 months if proper dosage is not provided. Due to deficiency, the infants start to experience multiple neurological symptoms like atrophy, anorexia, and impaired brain development. Due to impaired myelination, neural metabolism and neurotransmitter function, multiple development disorders are observed in children and infants. Many studies highlight the importance of nutrient especially vitamin B12 for proper brain development in infants. The vitamin B12 requirement continues from pre-birth period to school age as the brain is developing. If children do not get the required amount of vitamin B12 through lactation or food sources, it can result in limiting the brain development and impairment of myelination, peripheral nervous system, and neuron connectivity. The process of myelination and synthesizes of neurotransmitters starts from pregnancy and continues till 2 years, thus this period of life is crucial for brain development. Vitamin B12 deficiency during this period of life can impair the brain development and cognition process permanently. The damage to myelin during the brain development can have dire consequences for the central nervous system as it slows the process of conduction and communication with multiple systems. If nerve induction system is slowed, it can highly affect the learning and social communication ability of the child. Disruption of myelination during early years can lead to impaired cognition and atrophy which is sometime translated into neurological and behavioral abnormalities. The children who have faced vitamin B12 deficiency during the early years of life have impaired brain development and learning capability. Different studies conducted in school children showed that children who have adequate amount of vitamin B12 in their blood and ingest required amounts of the vitamin can perform better academically and have better learning capability. On the other hand, children who have reduced amount of animal based vitamins in their food or have vegetarian mothers have reduced cognition ability. Multiple studies have encountered reduce IQ level in children with vitamin B12 deficiency.

Chapter 3

3. Literature Review

The role of vitamins is described widely in a number of biochemical pathways that influence brain function. They play a crucial role as a coenzyme or cofactor and catalyze numerous important reactions in the body. Among all the other vitamins, B class of vitamins is a group of all water soluble vitamins that have a vital role in metabolism. Deficiency of vitamin B in body affects mental health of a person. Role of different types of vitamin B in mental health has been discussed in detail. This section will focus on presenting the evidence through literature studies and highlighting the importance of vitamin B group in maintaining brain health.

Schizophrenia is a severe mental disorder characterized by abnormal social behavior and an inability of separating real from unreal. Numerous studies have described the role of nutrients in maintaining the healthy mental health of a person. Research have demonstrated role of various vitamins in the development of schizophrenia. The symptoms of schizophrenia are well explained in the light of deficiencies of vitamins including vitamin B that leads to methylation deficits, oxidative damage, neuro degeneration that affects the brain development mechanisms and contribute to the onset of schizophrenia. A review article by Ramachandran and Thirunavakarasu gives a detailed overview of the role of vitamins in schizophrenia.[10] Most of the symptoms of schizophrenia are observed in people suffering from vitamin B deficiency and evidence supports the fact that symptoms improve with vitamin supplementation. The most important vitamin B discussed in reference to its association with schizophrenia is folic acid (vitamin B9). Folate deficiency can hinder the production of methyl donor and methylation of DNA and as a result it affects the expression of genes that are important in regulating neurodevelopmental processes. Moreover, deficiency of folic acid also obstructs the conversion of homocysteine to methionine and thereby results in the accretion of homocysteine that adversely effects the development of the brain in fetuses. A Mother deficient in folate and having high levels of homocysteine act as a risk factor for the development of schizophrenia. Furthermore, the study also explores the role of vitamin B12 in contribution to several neurologic problems. Seventy-eight percent of people suffering from schizophrenia were also having low levels of vitamin B12. Apart from this vitamin B3 (Niacin) is seen to have therapeutic effects in schizophrenia. The article successfully

---

[10] Ramachandran & Thirunavakarasu 2012:74-9.

demonstrates and proves the role of prenatal vitamin deficiency as a major factor that is responsible for the development of schizophrenia.

Another study by Herbison et al. (2012) explores the role of diet in the modulation of psychological well-being and the role of the vitamin B group in the production of neurotransmitters mainly serotonin. It further examines the relationship between vitamin B group and mental behavior of adolescents. It is a cross sectional analysis of the West Australian Pregnancy Cohort study. Food frequency questionnaires were collected and mental health was accessed using Youth Self Report (YSR) which measures behavior scores. Associations between mental health and vitamin B were analyzed using multiple linear regression method. Study results clearly suggested that low intake of vitamins B1, B2, B3, B5, B6 and B9 were responsible for high externalizing behavior scores. It was concluded that malnutrition contribute to the deficiency of vitamins that results in mental health problems in adolescence.[11]

A review study conducted by Harper titled "Thiamine (vitamin B1) deficiency and associated brain damage is still common throughout the world and prevention is safe and simple" discusses the role of vitamin B1

---

[11] Herbison, Hickling, Allen, O'Sullivan, Robinson, Bremner, & Oddy 2012: 634-638

in neurological and cardiac disorders. The literature highlights the fact that vitamin B1 deficiency is not limited to a specific region. Thiamine deficiency cases are reported from all over the world and many different population groups throughout the world are at the risk of developing severe cardiac and neurological disorders. People using alcohol are at high risk of developing mental disorders as alcohol destroys the stored vitamin B1 in the body. One of the most lethal disease caused by thiamine deficiency is Wernicke-Korsakoff syndrome which is a neurological disorder difficult to diagnose and in most of the cases remains undiagnosed. The study confirms that treatment with thiamine results in dramatic clinical improvements. Furthermore, it is suggested that thiamine status can be improved through consuming stable food products like flour etc.[12]

Another study titled *"vitamins and cognition"* published in 2011 reviews the role of vitamin supplementation in improving brain function. Vitamins play a vital role in maintaining the physiological and cellular processes of the body. Vitamins are directly related with the cognitive function and mood of an individual. Moreover, the study presents

---

[12] Harper 2006:1078-1082.

evidence regarding the importance of vitamin B among all the other vitamins in body and its importance in maintaining brain health.[13]

A study conducted by Malouf & Grimley aims at assessing the effectiveness of vitamin B supplementation in reducing the risk of developing cognitive impairment in older healthy individuals.[14] Vitamin B6 deficiency was found in almost every person suffering from cognitive decline and dementia. The study describes three chemically distinct compounds of vitamin B6 namely pyridoxal, pyrioxidine, and pyridoxamine that are involved in the regulation of brain function and mood. Vitamin B6 acts as a co-factor in the re-methylation of homocysteine. Therefore, deficiency of vitamin B6 is associated with increased level of homocysteine in blood which results in cerebrovascular disease and has toxic effects on neurons. Neuropsychiatric disorders including migraine, chronic pain, depression and seizures are directly linked to vitamin B6 deficiency. The study also confirms that deficiency of vitamin B6 is common in older adults.

---

[13] Kennedy & Haskell 2011:1957-1971.

[14] Malouf & Grimley Evans 2003.

The relationship between folic acid, vitamin B12 and the nervous system is also explored in a review study by Edward Reynolds. The author present numerous studies stating evidence that folic acid and vitamin B12 carry an intimate relationship among them and errors in their metabolism is associated with neuropathology and neuropsychiatric syndromes. The main role of these two vitamins is the conversion of homocysteine to methionine that is vital for genomic and non-genomic methylation and nucleotide synthesis. The study concludes that vitamin B12 and folic acid play key role in prevention of disorders of central nervous system, Alzheimer's disease, dementias and other mood related problems.

Another study titled *"Folate-vitamin B12 interaction in relation to cognitive impairment, anemia and biochemical indicators of vitamin B12 deficiency"* illustrates that high folate intake badly affects the natural history of vitamin B12 in elderly population. The study evaluated the interaction between low vitamin B12 levels and high serum folate with respect to cognitive impairment and anemia. Subjects demonstrated high levels of homocysteine circulating in the blood of patients having increased serum folate. Furthermore, it is also proved that high folate status is associated with impaired activity of vitamin B12 dependent enzymes namely, MMA coenzyme A mutase and methionine synthase.[15]

Study carried out by Maureen M. Black in 2011 titled "*Effects of vitamin B_{12} and folate deficiency on brain development in children*" identified the role of vitamin B12 for the brain development and cognition learning in children. This review study focuses on two mechanism of abnormal brain development; demyelination and inflammation that occur due to deficiency of vitamin B12. The children who were observed to be suffering from vitamin B12 deficiency shows symptoms like hypotonia, anorexia, liver enlargement and pigmentation. Infants breast feeding from vegetarian mothers are more prone to vitamin B12 deficiency and shows developmental impairment during the age of four to eleven months. Absence of intrinsic factor that is responsible for absorbing vitamin B12 from the food in mothers, a condition known as Pernicious anemia is considered one of the main reason of developmental abnormalities in infants. During a case study presented in the paper, similar developmental impairments are observed among infants of vegetarian mothers as well as pernicious anemia. The infants of both groups showed delayed and reduced cognitive ability and brain development. Reduced level of

---

[15] Selhub, Morris, Jacques & Rosenberg 2009:702S-706S.

vitamin B12 in infants results in restricting the process of myelination and changes in tissue levels of different neurotransmitters causing alteration in neurological metabolism and anatomical system. During the early year of brain development when rate of growth is maximum, the vitamin B12 deficiency result in destruction of neuron myelin and condition known as atrophy. The demyelination effect the synapse and conduction system in brain resulting in behavioral abnormalities. The vitamin B12 deficiency is common in infants and mothers in societies with minimal consumption animal food. The study carried out in Boston schools suggested low IQ level and reduced cognition ability in children who have poorer vitamin B12 diet in earlier years. This review study has great significance in showing the adverse effects of vitamin B12 deficiency on the cognition and brain development. Similarly the deficiency in later years has been observed to be a source of depression in adults.

Another study conducted by Selhub, Bagley, Miller and Rosenberg (2000) "*B vitamins, homocysteine, and neurocognitive function in the elderly*" shows the importance of vitamin B6, vitamin B9 and vitamin B12 for normal neurological function by playing significant roles in one carbon metabolism. Deficiency in these vitamins results in impairment of psychological function and associated with multiple neurological disorders. In the study, it is indicated that with age, the ability to absorb vitamin B12 from food become limited due to decreased secretion of intrinsic factor. Another important factor is increased bacterial growth due to atrophic gastritis condition as bacterial colonies take up the vitamin B12. The thinking and memory test conducted in the study showed that individuals having low concentration of folic acid, riboflavin and vitamin B12 performed poorly in these test showing the effect of vitamins on cognitive function. After using vitamins as supplements, the test scores had improved to a greater extent. The association between vitamin levels and cognitive function is established through one-carbon metabolism. Thus pathway is characterized by the generation of methionine which is crucial product for the brain cells. The folic acid, riboflavin and vitamin B12 act as important cofactors for this pathway. The large portion of methionine produced in converted into *S*-adenosylmethionine (SAM) by ATP, which is responsible for the production of neurotransmitters and myelin. One possibility presented for the impaired cognitive and neurological function is reduced methylation in brain tissue. The increased level of homocysteine in blood plasma is an indicator of inadequate vitamin B status mainly folic acid, Riboflavin and vitamin B12. During a carried out by Riggs *et al.,* (1996) a cognitive ability test is carried out on males aging from 58 years to 80 years. Lower level of folate and vitamin B12 indicated poorer results in these test. However, the level of homocysteine were relatively higher than normal levels indicating the inverse relation with vitamin levels. Studies have also indicated the prevalent depression symptoms in individuals with elevated homocysteine level which may be due to decreased vitamin B12 and folate level.

A study "*Vitamin B12 deficiency and depression in physically disabled older women: epidemiological evidence from the Women's Health and Aging Study*" by Pennix *et al.,* (2014) aim to prove the hypothesis that appropriate level of folate and vitamin B12 is necessary for the integrity and development of neurological system.[16] For this purpose, epidemiological study has been conducted on older women to investigate the association of folate and vitamin B12 levels on depression. The women were tested for plasma level of folate, homocysteine and vitamin B12 and through geriatric scale for depression, categorized for extent of neurological depression. The geriatric scale values lied in the interval of 0-30 with higher values indicate extreme depression. The value is measured on the basis of occurrence of different symptom of depression.

---

[16] Penninx, Guralnik, Ferrucci, Fried, Allen, & Stabler 2014.

Statistical analysis is carried out on different proportions to find the association between vitamin deficiency and occurrence of depression in test subjects. In the study, it was discovered 27% of the depressed women were also observed to be suffering from deficiency of folate and vitamin B12. According to the results 40% of the women with high scores on depression scale have vitamin levels below the threshold value that is set on 258 pmol/liter. Through analysis it was conferred that vitamin deficiency is more prevalent in women who were suffering from symptoms of severe and mild depression than women who were not showing any signs of depression. Regression model of the data indicated that higher association level is found between vitamin B12 and folate deficiency and severe symptoms of depression in women included in the study. The risk of developing depression in elder women who are suffering from vitamin deficiency is two times greater than women not having any vitamin deficiency. The depressed subjects were observed to have high levels of different metabolites like methylmalonic acid which is observed to be linked with the development of depression. Similarly the inhibition of synthesis of *S*-adenosylmethionine due to deficiency of vitamin B12 is also considered one of the reasons for the symptoms of depression.

A case study presented by Berry, Sagar and Tripathi (2003) titled *"Catatonia and other psychiatric symptoms with vitamin B12 deficiency"* also focuses on the neurological consequences of deficiency of vitamin B12.[17] In the study, a case of 52 years old female patient who was suffering from depression, cognitive dysfunction and psychosis. The plasma screening indicated the reduced level of cobalamin or vitamin B12 in the patient due to a complete vegetarian diet for many years. The study suggested that prolonged deficiency of vitamin B12 and neurological symptoms are difficult to treat as long periods of deficiency can induce irreversible damage to axons. In the study, it was identified that vitamin B12 deficiency was overlooked in many psychiatric and neurological disorders as clinical symptoms of depression and psychosis is rarely accepted to be a reason from dietary deficiencies. Due to the inability to identify the involvement of vitamin B12 deficiency in psychiatric symptoms result in the worsening of the situation until the condition becomes completely irreversible. The difficulty with neurological disorders is the small window of treatment time in which the adverse effect on brain tissues and neurological system can be rectified. The

---

[17] Berry, Sagar & Tripathi 2003:156-159.

persistence of condition can induce irreversible damage in the brain cells and become source to a cascade of neurological problems. Another problem identified in clinical treatment of neurological disorders is unawareness of the high prevalence of vitamin B12 deficiency in most patients. It was identified that 31% patients of cognitive impairment and 12% of the depressed patients were associated with vitamin B12 deficiency. The authors suggested that the case presented in the study provide evidence for the importance of screening for the level of vitamin B12 in different psychiatric patients so as to detect the dietary deficiencies at earlier stages.

Another case study presented by Milanlıoğlu, A. (2011) focused on a female patient of 33 years old suffering from the symptoms of fatigue, sleeplessness, psychological disinterest, sadness and rapid loss of weight. Upon investigation, major dietary source are identified to be plant source food. Over the last few years, her psychological condition had worsen with occurrence of additional symptoms of irritability and aggression. She also faced difficulty in communication and movements. During clinical investigation, hormones and blood count were within normal range but the levels of vitamin B12 is observed to be 82 pg/mL as compared to normal level which should be from 200 to 900 pg/ml. She was suffering from deficiency of vitamin B12 which induced the symptoms of depression and psychological deterioration. She was treated with supplements of vitamin B12 which improved the mental health to great extent. After one month of therapy, most of the psychological symptoms either disappeared or reduced to a manageable level. The vegetarian mode of diet has played important role in developing vitamin B12 deficiency in body and hence mental health deterioration. It was also identified that different anti-depressant agents fail to perform functions if vitamin deficiency persist. In many patients who were suffering from different neurological disorders specially depression, the therapeutic agents did not show any effect until combined with vitamin B12 treatment. In many clinical cases, the vitamin treatment alone is sufficient to reduce the symptoms of depression and mental impairment.

A study conducted by Robert, Langan, Kimberly and Zawstoski also addresses the role of cobalamin (vitamin B12) deficiency in development of psychiatric symptoms and anemia.[18] The study also provide evidence for the increased level of homocysteine as a result of vitamin B12 deficiency. Authors provide recommendations that screening

---

[18] Langan & Zawistoski 2011:1425-1430.

of blood serum for vitamin B12 deficiency should be carried out by all physicians for high as well as low risk individuals so as to identify the problem at earlier stage. Moreover, patients should be screened for the level of homocysteine and methylmalonic acid as these metabolites also pose a threat to brain developmental and can trigger psychiatric symptoms. The normal dosage of vitamin B12 deficient patient provided in the study is injecting 1 mg intramuscularly up to 8 weeks and in some cases 1 mg injection has to be maintained for whole life. But the neurological disorders that result due to deficiency of vitamin B12 may not get treated solely from vitamin treatment, as brain cells have endured damage due to low level of vitamin B12. The amount of vitamin B12 absorbed from food gets reduced as individual cross age limit of fifty years. As the intrinsic factor started to reduce in the body, less amount of vitamin B12 is absorbed from food. So study recommended that individuals above the age of 50 must include crystalline supplements of vitamin b12 and fortified vitamin B12 food in their daily routine to meet the requirements of the vitamin in the body. Similarly, vegetarian populations also have to obtain vitamin B12 through the supplements to avoid the deficiencies. The author suggested that elder population must be routinely assessed for the vitamin B12 levels as well as homocysteine levels to detect the risk of neurological disorder. In case of mental health deterioration along with anti-depressant and other neurological agents, vitamin B12 treatment must also be prescribed.

Another review study conducted by Roy, Sher & Adams (2012) also provides evidence for the association of Vitamin B12 with the development of depression. A demographic study was carried out on 278 patients who were categorized as depressed according to the criteria provided by DSM-IV. Through analysis it was concluded that 70% of the test subjects who were suffering from depression and other psychiatric disorders have been deficient in vitamin B12 level. Multiple studies identified that the role of vitamin B12 treatment in increasing the efficiency of anti-depressant agents. The author concluded that there have been enough evidences for the involvement of vitamin B12 deficiency in developing psychological symptoms as well as for the assistive role of vitamin treatment with psychotherapy. However, fewer studies provide evidence that vitamin B12 therapy alone have preventive and cure capabilities in different neurological disorders.

Chapter 4

4. Recommendations

As the body lacks the ability to store vitamin B for long period of time, thus these have to be ingested on daily basis to avoid deficiency in the body. All the water soluble vitamins especially vitamin B complex is required in low quantities so its requirement can easily be fulfilled from food. To avoid adverse effect of vitamin B deficiency on mental health as well as physical health, it is very necessary to consume a balance diet. As mentioned earlier that vitamin B deficiency is prevalent in populations and individuals who keep on consuming just plant source food. To meet the daily requirement vitamin B in the body, both the animal and plant source must be incorporated in the diet. The vitamin B is required in very low amount which can easily be obtained from food. The following is given the amount of Vitamin B required by the body:

- Vitamin B1: required amount per day in adult male 1.2 milligrams and adult female 1.1 milligrams.
- Vitamin B2: required amount per day in adult male 1.3 milligrams and adult female 1.1 milligrams.

- Vitamin B3: required amount per day in adult male 16 milligrams and adult female 14 milligrams
- Vitamin B5: required amount per day in adult male 5 milligrams and adult female 5 milligrams
- Vitamin B6: required amount per day in adult male 1.3 milligrams and adult female 1.3-1.5 milligrams.
- Vitamin B7: required amount per day in adult male and female is 0.04 milligrams (40 micrograms).
- Vitamin B9: required amount per day in adult male 0.4 milligrams and adult female 0.4 milligrams
- Vitamin B12: required amount in adult male and female is 0.0024 milligrams (2.4 microgram).[19]

Above mentioned requirements can easily be met from food including vegetables, whole grains and meat. The dairy and poultry products must be important part of diet along with vegetables and fruit so as to obtain the balance energy content. Pregnant and lactating women specially need to monitor the daily consumption of Vitamin B complex so as to ensure normal brain development in children. Most of the medical professionals prescribe different vitamin supplements to pregnant and lactating women

---

[19] Acu-cell.com, 2015

to avoid any kind of deficiency. These supplements must be supported by a balanced and healthy diet to maintain the required levels of Vitamin B in the body. Similarly in early years of life, children have rapid brain and body development thus extensively need to fulfill their vitamin requirement to avoid the development of any mental and neurological disorder. With age, the ability to absorb the vitamin B from food reduces due to which deficiencies are more prevalent in elderly population. So it is very necessary to monitor the plasma level of water soluble vitamins and take proper vitamin B supplements prescribed by a medical professional to avoid development of mental illness. Patients who have been identified with vitamin B deficiency needs to fulfill the deficient amount through supplement therapies that include intramuscular, intranasal and oral uptake of vitamin B supplements. The intramuscular therapy method has shown the most success rate in vitamin B deficient patients but oral ingestion of supplements tablets is also a very reliable method. Patients of different neurological and developmental disorders must be tested for serum levels of vitamin B to identify the deficiencies in earlier stage so that it can be rectified with prescribed supplement treatments which also have positive effects on mental health. Chapter 5

5. Conclusion

Vitamins are essential to the normal functioning of our body just like other minerals and nutrients. They usually serve individual purposes or mainly act as cofactors to facilitate various biochemical reactions in our body. One of the most essential and vital group of vitamins is vitamin B complex that makeup the nutritional powerhouse. This key vitamin group plays an important role in regulating bodily functions, mental health and various cognitive processes and provide mental stability and emotional balance for the wholeness of man. Therefore, it can be said that vitamin B complex is required in every important biochemical process taking place in our body. Mortality rate associated with the severe deficiency of vitamin B is high in which it is mainly involved in regulating the central nervous system. Malnutrition or too much use of alcohol reduces the amount of vitamin B in our body and leads to serious disorders including Wernicke-Korsakoff syndrome, schizophrenia, Alzheimer's, dementia, memory loss, Beriberi, and other mental health problems. The facts and figures presented in the study suggest that daily intake of vitamin B must be regularly monitored and that care must be taken especially in pregnant and lactating women as vitamin B9 is crucial to the normal brain functioning of fetus. Furthermore, the brain and central nervous system development is taking place mainly in the early years of childhood; therefore, mothers should be well focused in giving their child diet enriched in vitamins. The present study has clearly demonstrated the role of vitamin B in mental health and has provided recommendations so as to improve the vitamin B status in the wholeness of man.

Chapter 6

6. References

Acu-cell.com., (2015). *B-Vitamins: DRI/RDA, Overdose, Side Effects, Deficiency Symptoms.* Retrieved 22 June 2015, from <http://www.acu-cell.com/bx2.html>

Ball, G. F. (2008). *Vitamins: their role in the human body.* John Wiley & Sons.

Berry, N., Sagar, R., & Tripathi, B. M. (2003). Catatonia and other psychiatric symptoms with vitamin B12 deficiency. *Acta Psychiatrica Scandinavica, 108*(2), 156-159.

Black, M. M. (2008). Effects of vitamin B12 and folate deficiency on brain development in children. *Food and nutrition bulletin, 29*(2 Suppl), S126.

Cooper, J. R., & Pincus, J. H. (1979). The role of thiamine in nervous tissue. *Neurochemical research, 4*(2), 223-239.

Harper, C. (2006). Thiamine (vitamin B1) deficiency and associated brain damage is still common throughout the world and prevention is simple and safe! *European Journal of Neurology, 13*(10), 1078-1082.

Herbison, C. E., Hickling, S., Allen, K. L., O'Sullivan, T. A., Robinson, M., Bremner, A. P., ... & Oddy, W. H. (2012). Low intake of B-vitamins is associated with poor adolescent mental health and behaviour. *Preventive medicine*, *55*(6), 634-638.

Jacob, R. A., & Swendseid, M. E. (1996). Niacin. *Present knowledge in nutrition*, 184-190.

Kennedy, D. O., & Haskell, C. F. (2011). Vitamins and cognition. *Drugs*, *71*(15), 1957-1971.

Langan, R. C., & Zawistoski, K. J. (2011). Update on vitamin B12 deficiency. American family physician, 83(12), 1425-1430.

Malouf, R., & Grimley Evans, J. (2003). Vitamin B6 for cognition. *Cochrane Database Syst Rev*, *4*.

Milanlıoğlu, A. (2011). Vitamin B12 deficiency and depression. *Journal of Clinical and Experimental Investigations*, *2*(4).

NOVEUP, G. D. (1953). Metabolic functions of pantothenic acid.

Penninx, B. W., Guralnik, J. M., Ferrucci, L., Fried, L. P., Allen, R. H., & Stabler, S. P. (2014). Vitamin B12 deficiency and depression in physically disabled older women: epidemiologic evidence from the Women's Health and Aging Study. *American Journal of Psychiatry*.

Ramachandran, P., & Thirunavakarasu, P. (2012). Vitamins in schizophrenia: a literature review. *Andhra Pradesh Journal Of Psychological Medicine*, *13*(2), 74-9. Retrieved from http://journaldatabase.info/articles/vitamins_schizophrenia_literature.html

Riggs, K. M., Spiro, A. I. I. I., Tucker, K., & Rush, D. (1996). Relations of vitamin B-12, vitamin B-6, folate, and homocysteine to cognitive performance in the Normative Aging Study. *The American journal of clinical nutrition*, *63*(3), 306-314.

Roy, H., Sher, A., & Adams, S. (2012). Vitamin B12 and Depression. *Journal of Pharmacy and Alternative Medicine*, *2*, 9-12.

Sauve, A. A. (2008). NAD+ and vitamin B3: from metabolism to therapies. *Journal of Pharmacology and Experimental Therapeutics*, *324*(3), 883-893.

Selhub, J., Bagley, L. C., Miller, J., & Rosenberg, I. H. (2000). B vitamins, homocysteine, and neurocognitive function in the elderly. *The American journal of clinical nutrition, 71*(2), 614s-620s.

Selhub, J., Morris, M. S., Jacques, P. F., & Rosenberg, I. H. (2009). Folate–vitamin B-12 interaction in relation to cognitive impairment, anemia, and biochemical indicators of vitamin B-12 deficiency. *The American journal of clinical nutrition, 89*(2), 702S-706S.

Spector, H., Maass, A. R., Michaud, L., Elvehjem, C. A., & Hart, E. B. (1943). The role of riboflavin in blood regeneration. *Journal of Biological Chemistry, 150*(1), 75-87.

Tahiliani, A. G., & Beinlich, C. J. (1990). Pantothenic acid in health and disease. *Vitamins and hormones, 46*, 165-228.

Von Muralt, A. (1958). The role of thiamine (vitamin B1) in nervous excitation. *Experimental cell research, 14*(Suppl 5), 72.

Thank you for your continued support:

Facebook:
https://www.facebook.com/drgilliamlovesnaturalsolutions?ref=bookmarks

Email: drtiffany.gilliam@gmail.com

Dr. Tiffany Gilliam, N.D., MH, CNC, CHS